MANOJ PRASAD

Manoj the Yogi on Kriya Yoga

A Guide to Awaken the Chakras and Kundalini

To
Swami Satyananda Saraswati and Paramahansa Yogananda
who showed me the way
and to all my supporters
who lifted me up

All my love and gratitude
Manoj the Yogi

Contents

Copyright Permissions

The images of a watercolor background[1] (cover), a human spine[2] and an arrow head[3] (introduction) were provided by freepik.com[4] and have been used in accordance with their license.

[1] https://www.freepik.com/free-vector/abstract-decorative-watercolor-background_9783887.htm

[2] https://www.freepik.com/free-vector/sketches-human-spine_843085.htm

[3] https://www.freepik.com/free-vector/flat-design-arrow-collection_5940015.htm

[4] https://www.freepik.com/

Introduction

Welcome to my book on Kriya Yoga! I'm so happy and thankful that you've decided to read it and I hope you'll find it beneficial.

I believe we are spiritual beings and the purpose of life is spiritual development. I believe that everyone is experiencing spiritual development every day, and the only difference is the rate of development that is occurring. This book is for those seeking to increase their rate of spiritual development.

Accelerated spiritual development is accomplished by awakening the chakras and then the kundalini. Chakras are spiritual energy centers in the body connected by energy pathways. Kundalini is powerful spiritual energy that enters the body at the Root Chakra located in the coccyx (tailbone) and travels up the spine and out through the top of the head.

The practice of Kriya Yoga allows one to awaken the chakras and kundalini, and achieve accelerated spiritual development in an easy and efficient manner. This has been nicely summed up by Paramahansa Yogananda in the book " Autobiography of a Yogi"[5] (Chapter 26) as follows:

> *The* Kriya Yogi *mentally directs his life energy to revolve, upward and downward, around the six spinal centers (medullary, cervical, dorsal, lumbar, sacral, and coccygeal plexuses) which correspond to the twelve astral signs of the zodiac, the symbolic Cosmic Man. One-half minute of revolution of energy around the sensitive spinal cord of man effects subtle progress in his evolution; that half-minute of Kriya equals one*

---

[5] https://www.ananda.org/autobiography/

year of natural spiritual unfoldment.

As you can see, it's possible to accelerate one's spiritual development by many orders of magnitude with Kriya Yoga. However, to fully realize this benefit, I feel that integrating this technique into a complete yoga practice produces the best results. Many Kriya Yoga schools point to the Hatha Yoga Pradipika[6] as the primary source for accomplishing this.

This scripture is broken in four parts:

1. Asanas (physical postures)
2. Pranayama (breathing practices)
3. Mudras (seals or locks)
4. Samadhi (self realization)

I'll talk about each of these parts, but let's start at the end and then see how we get there. So what is samadhi or self realization? On page 154, it is stated that:

> As salt being dissolved in water becomes one with it, so when Atma and mind become one, it is called Samadhi.

Atma is the soul or true self, and the analogy is a perfect one, as salt does not instantly dissolve in water, it takes time and happens slowly bit by bit, but we can speed up the process with a bit of stirring.

Samadhi happens most often when the body has been still for some time, and while the mind has remained empty but aware. This is the practice of meditation, and while it's simple to describe, it can be difficult to perform. We've put the salt in the water, but we can't sit still and thoughts keep entering our mind, so the salt doesn't dissolve.

This is where those previous three parts now enter the picture. The ability

---

[6] https://archive.org/details/HathaYogaPradipika-
      SanskritTextWithEnglishTranslationAndNotes/mode/2up

to sit motionless for extended periods of time requires a fit and flexible body. This is achieved by practicing various physical movements, stretches and postures (part 1). The ability to still our mind for extended periods of time is greatly enhanced by developing awareness of our breathing through breathing practices (part 2). Finally, the ability to merge with the Atma, and give the water some good continuous stirring, is greatly enhanced with breath retention combined with mudras or locks (part 3).

In fact, all three parts contribute to the stirring as they all have an effect on the chakras and kundalini. The postures have a subtle effect, while breath awareness has a stronger effect, but breath retention with locks has the strongest effect of all in awakening the chakras and kundalini, which in turn bring the Atma to the surface to merge with the mind.

The levels of samadhi that can be experienced are many, but ultimately you're now on a journey where one day you'll realize yourself as an immortal being of infinite love.

Course Overview

My goal for this book is to start with something that is suitable for all ages at all levels of ability and then provide options for more advanced practice based on physical ability and spiritual readiness.

I feel the basic Kriya Yoga technique, introduced in the previous section and described in detail in the next, is suitable for all ages as it allows for a passive and safe awakening of the chakras as presented in the early lessons. I call this practice Kriya Breathing in the course with locks added in later lessons. This practice is also known as Kriya Proper or Kriya Pranayama.

There are two other core Kriya Yoga techniques that I include in this course which I call Forward Bending Breathing (maha mudra) and Face Fingers Breathing (bhramari). The first practice is well known by all schools as Maha Mudra, but the second practice is more popularly known as Yoni Mudra or Yoti Mudra, and does not include humming as Bhramari does. I personally find the Bhramari variation of this practice the most beneficial so that's the one I've included. With both practices I start with basic versions and then introduce intermediate and advanced versions as the lessons progress.

The postures presented should be achievable for most people, and represent the minimum required for achieving the necessary level of fitness and flexibility. In terms of breathing practices, the Kriya Yoga techniques mostly have this covered, but there are two techniques I feel complement the Kriya techniques which I've included: Alternate Nostril Breathing (nadi shodhana) and Rapid Belly Breathing (bhastrika). Finally, both Breath and Chakra Meditation practices are presented with their respective uses and benefits explained.

Lesson 1

- Ocean Breathing (ujjayi)
- Alternate Nostril Breathing (with Ocean Breathing)
- Kriya Breathing (with Ocean Breathing)
- Face Fingers Breathing (with Ocean Breathing)
- Breath Meditation (with Normal Breathing)

Lesson 2

- Basic Asana (Lying Down Stretch, Lower Back Massage, Ankle Rotation, Squat Pose, Tiptoe Pose)
- Accomplished Pose (siddhasana)
- Forward Bending Breathing (with Ocean Breathing)

Lesson 3

- Intermediate Asana (Sun Salutation, Corpse Pose, Spinal Twist)
- Abdominal Lock (uddiyana bandha)
- Rapid Belly Breathing (with both nostrils)

Lesson 4

- Alternate Nostril Breathing (breath retention added)
- Rapid Belly Breathing (single nostril added)
- Kriya Breathing (double rounds)
- Forward Bending Breathing (breath retention added)
- Face Fingers Breathing (breath retention added)
- Third Eye Meditation

Lesson 5

- Basic Locks (Third Eye Lock, Nose Tip Lock, Basic Tongue Lock, Root Lock)
- Alternate Nostril Breathing (basic locks added)
- Rapid Belly Breathing (basic locks added)
- Kriya Breathing (basic locks added)
- Forward Bending Breathing (basic locks added)
- Face Fingers Breathing (basic locks added)
- Chakra Meditation

Lesson 6

- Intermediate Locks (Throat Lock, Solar Lock, Navel Lock, Sacral Lock)
- Alternate Nostril Breathing (throat/solar locks added)
- Forward Bending Breathing (throat/navel locks added)
- Face Fingers Breathing (sacral lock added)

Lesson 7

- Advanced Tongue Lock Preparation (Tongue Clicking, Frenulum Stretch, Full Face Stretch)
- Advanced Tongue Lock (khechari mudra)
- Kriya Breathing (try "up the spine" if you haven't yet)

Spiritual Anatomy

In this section we will dive into the details of our spiritual anatomy, including the chakras, pathways (nadis), and chakra activation points (kshetrams) or APs for short. So what are APs? These are points on the surface of the body that when we concentrate on, or move our concentration through them, it creates a sensation which passes through the nerves to the chakra itself. These APs are mirrored on the front and back of the body, but in general the position of the front AP or FAP defines the position of the chakra in the spine and the position of the back AP or BAP as well.

- The Root Chakra (muladhara) is located in the coccyx region of the spine. Its FAP is located at the perineum for men and at the cervix for women. It has no BAP.
- The Sacral Chakra (swadhisthana) is located in the sacral region of the spine across from its FAP at the pubic symphysis. Its BAP is directly behind that.
- The Navel Chakra (manipura) is located in the lumbar region of the spine across from its FAP at the navel. Its BAP is directly behind that.
- The Solar Chakra (hrit/surya) is located where the lumbar and thoracic regions of the spine meet across from its FAP at the diaphragm. Its BAP is directly behind that.
- The Heart Chakra (anahata) is located in the thoracic region of the spine across from its FAP at the sternum. Its BAP is directly behind that.
- The Throat Chakra (vishuddhi) is located in the cervical region of the spine across from its FAP at the thyroid. Its BAP is directly behind that.
- The Third Eye Chakra (ajna) is located in the center of the head across from its FAP (bhrumadhya) at the eyebrow center. Its BAP (medulla) is directly behind that.
- The Crown Chakra (sahasrara) is located just below the top of the head. Its FAP is located at bregma and its BAP (bindu) is located at the top back of the head.

Here's a diagram of these eight chakras in the spine and head along with their FAPs and BAPs connected by dotted lines.

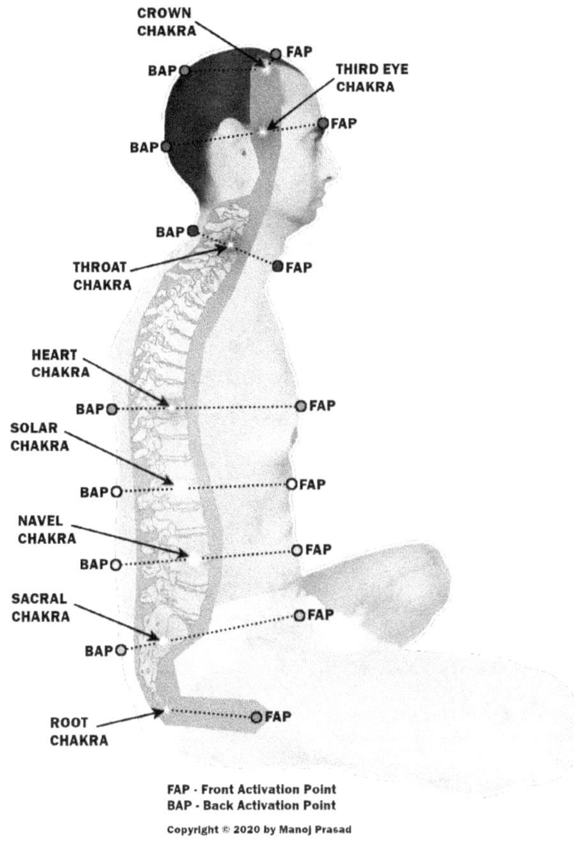

Chakras

For those already familiar with the chakras, the above list and diagram may look a bit odd. In P. Yogananda's quote above he mentions the lumbar plexus (navel) and the dorsal plexus (heart), but not the solar plexus. This is typical in eastern spirituality, but for those raised in western spirituality, they are familiar with the sacral plexus and the solar plexus but not the lumbar plexus. However, in both systems they do acknowledge these other chakras as existing, but refer to them as being secondary rather than primary. I've chosen to include both as both are used in my practices.

Also, every nerve plexus in the body corresponds to a chakra, so there are far more than the few I've listed here, and there's one more I make use of in these practices which is called the Palate Chakra (lalana) and it is located in the soft palate.

Revolving the Energy

There are basically two ways for revolving the energy around the body. In the first method we simply reinforce the natural flow of energy in the body which goes up the front and down the spine. We exhale fully and concentrate at the Root FAP then begin inhaling while moving our concentration up past the Sacral FAP, Navel FAP, etc. until the Throat FAP, finally through our head to the Crown BAP as our inhalation completes. After that, we begin our exhalation and downward movement of our concentration through the Third Eye Chakra, Throat Chakra, etc. until the Root Chakra before returning to the Root FAP where we started as our exhalation completes and we're ready to start the next revolution.

Here's a diagram showing this pathway.

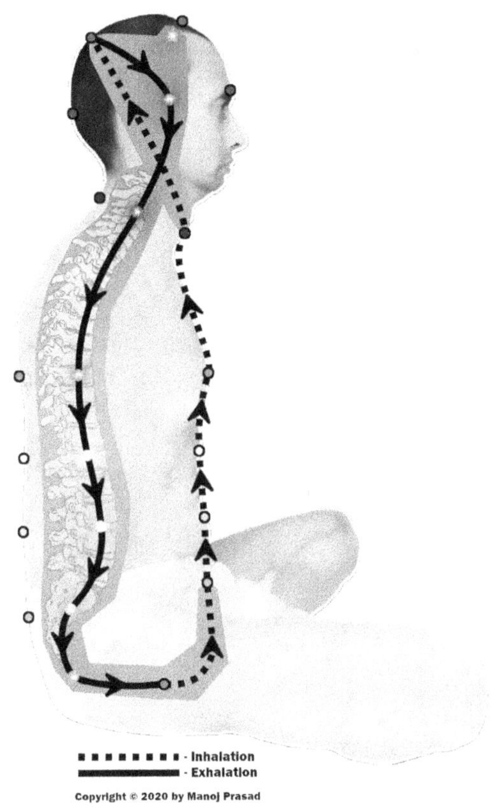

Down the Spine Breathing

If you're an absolute beginner, then I recommend using this direction of revolution until you're able to feel the energy moving through your body, along with tingling sensations at the FAPs and chakras, as well as changing colors in your vision when your eyes are closed. The purpose of this first method is to awaken the chakras, and these experiences indicate that this is happening. There are an infinite number of spiritual experiences that are possible, but these are the most common.

The purpose of the second method is to awaken the kundalini, and as mentioned at the start, kundalini energy moves up the spine which is in the opposite direction from the natural flow of energy down the spine. Our goal now becomes to reverse the flow of energy in the spine by going against the flow which is much more difficult compared to going with the flow. The obvious analogy is like trying to paddle upstream against the current in a kayak or canoe.

We again exhale fully and start at the Root FAP but this time as we inhale we move our concentration to the Root Chakra and up the spine past the Sacral Chakra, Navel Chakra, etc. until the Third Eye Chakra, finally over to the Third Eye FAP as our inhalation completes. After that, we begin our exhalation and moving our concentration up over the top of our head past the Crown FAP and BAP, then down past the Third Eye BAP, Throat BAP, etc. until the Sacral BAP then down to the Root Chakra and back over to the Root FAP where we started as our exhalation completes and we're ready to start the next revolution.

Here's a diagram showing this pathway.

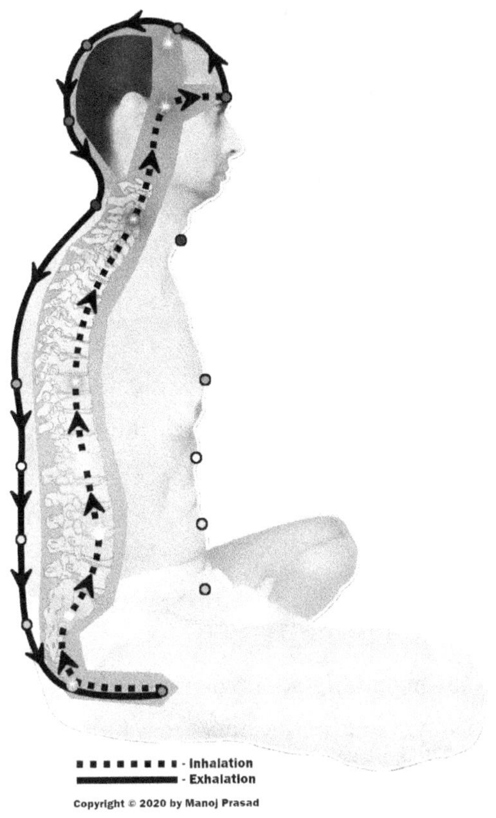

Up the Spine Breathing

This second method is completely optional and is only for those interested in reaching more advanced stages of spiritual development. If you're an absolute beginner, you can try this method and see what effect it has, and if you experience good results then feel free to continue with it, but in general, beginners have better success with the first method as it is much easier to go with the natural flow of energy down the spine than trying to reverse it.

The lessons that follow can be done with either direction of revolution depending where you are in your spiritual development and what your goals are. I will simply use the words "inhale up the body" and "exhale down the body" to mean either:

- Inhale up the front passage then exhale down the spinal passage for chakra awakening, or…
- Inhale up the spinal passage then exhale over the head and down the back for kundalini awakening.

In general, I would recommend using the "down the spine" direction for at least a few months before trying the "up the spine" direction.

General Guidelines

The following guidelines will help maximize the effectiveness of your practice:

- Practice every day at the same time in the same spot, but any time or spot is fine.
- Practice before breakfast, but before any meal or before sleeping is fine.

As you progress through the lessons, you may notice that you start to interpret life in a different way. For example, there may be a particular food that you've always enjoyed, then you notice that it has stopped tasting as good and you find yourself enjoying something else that you never liked before. This is normal and it simply means you've evolved beyond one particular food to another.

Essentially, your senses, both physical (smell, taste, etc.) and non-physical (intuitive, psychic, etc.) will guide you as required. For quickest progress, it helps to make your rational mind subordinate to these other senses and just go where they lead you.

Finally, make sure you're having fun every step of the way!

Lesson 1: Basic Kriya

The process of breathing may involve three different body movements.

- Pulling the diaphragm downward to pull air into the lowest part of the lungs.
- Expanding the chest outward to pull air into the central part of the lungs.
- Pushing the collarbones upward to pull air into the upper part of the lungs.

It is highly recommended to practice "diaphragm first" breathing at all times no matter what activity you are engaged in, but especially for these practices. The term "diaphragm first" means that you always inhale using your diaphragm first as much as you can, before using anything else. You expand your belly before you expand your chest which should not even be required most of the time.

For all the practices I've included in this book, all the breathing is done through the nose with the mouth closed.

This lesson is suitable for all ages with the only requirement being the ability to sit up and move your arms while sitting in a chair or on the ground. Also, feel free to use a cushion or stool to make yourself comfortable. Don't lean back against anything, instead hold your head high to create a slight inward curve at the lower back.

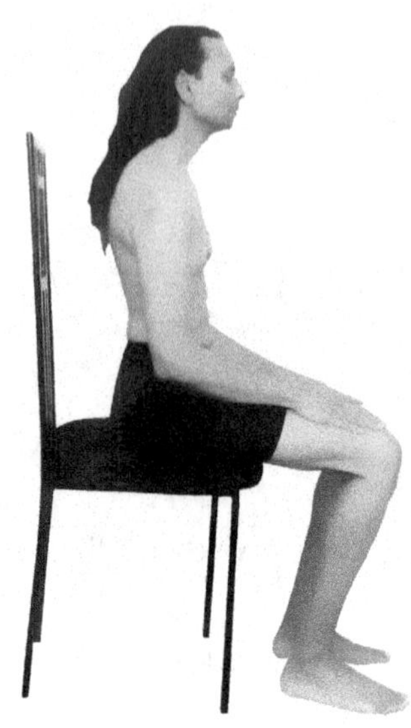

Ocean Breathing (ujjayi)

Ocean breathing is performed by applying a slight constriction to the throat causing a slight noise to be heard when breathing, which sounds like the waves from a distant ocean. The constriction applied is the same as when whispering or trying to fog up a window. Try one deep diaphragm breath using ocean breathing. All of the slow deep breathing practices are done with ocean breathing, and only meditation uses normal silent breathing.

Alternate Nostril Breathing (nadi shodhana)

Alternate nostril breathing involves closing one nostril and breathing through the other. The entire practice is done with ocean breathing. Each nostril is connected to a spiritual pathway (ida and pingala nadis), and by closing one nostril we force spiritual energy through the other pathway. This helps activate, purify and balance the flow of energy in these pathways.

1. Exhale fully and close your eyes, then use your right thumb to close your

right nostril and inhale fully through your left nostril.

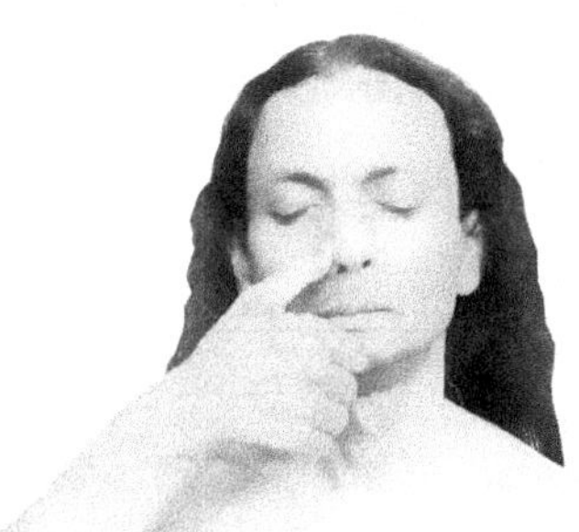

2. Release your right nostril and use your middle and ring fingers to close your left nostril and exhale fully through your right nostril.

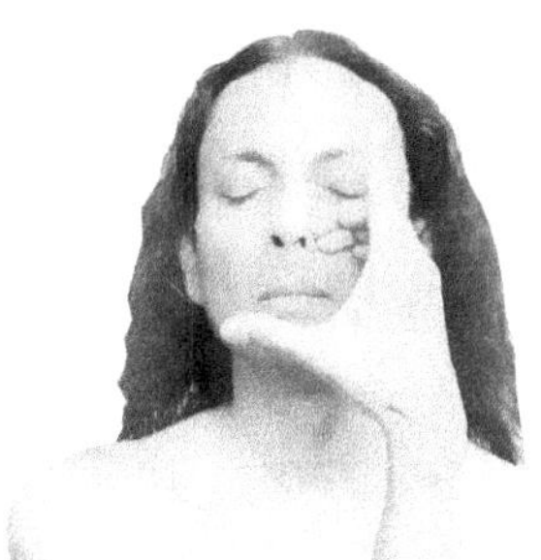

3. Keep your left nostril closed and inhale fully through your right nostril.
4. Release your left nostril and use your thumb to close your right nostril and exhale fully through your left nostril.
5. Release both nostrils, concentrate on the Root FAP and inhale up the body to the top AP (Crown BAP or Third Eye FAP) then exhale down the body to the Root FAP.

This completes 1 round. Perform rounds for 1 to 2 minutes. If you have learned a different hand position for this practice, feel free to use that.

The goal is to slow down your breathing such that each inhale and exhale lasts for approximately 12-15 seconds and only one round is performed. The following table provides an example progression. Note that "Week" in the table could easily be "Day" or "Month" depending on your ability.

Week	Inhale/Exhale (sec)	Rounds (1-2 min)
1	4-6	3
2	7-10	2
3	11-20	1

Alternate Nostril Breathing Progression

Kriya Breathing

This is the main practice that was described in the introduction. It involves simply inhaling up the body and exhaling down the body in continuous revolutions with ocean breathing.

1. Exhale fully and close your eyes, concentrate on the Root FAP and inhale up the body to the top AP (Crown BAP or Third Eye FAP) then exhale down the body to the Root FAP.

This completes 1 round. Perform rounds for 6 minutes.

Once you're able to extend each inhale and exhale to about 15 seconds, then each round will take 30 seconds, so 12 rounds can be completed in 6 minutes. An easy way to count 12 rounds is by using the segments on your fingers and moving your thumb through the segments to track your progress.

Start by touching your thumb to the tip of your index finger for the first round, then at the start of the second round move to the middle segment of your index finger and so on through all 3 segments on all 4 fingers for a total of 12 segments and 12 rounds.

Face Fingers Breathing (bhramari)

Face fingers breathing involves placing your fingers on your face and exhaling with a humming sound. This practice helps awaken psychic sensitivity to spiritual energy.

The thumbs go in your ears, the index and middle fingers on your eyes, the ring fingers on your nose next to the middle fingers (leaving the nostrils open), and the little fingers on your lips.

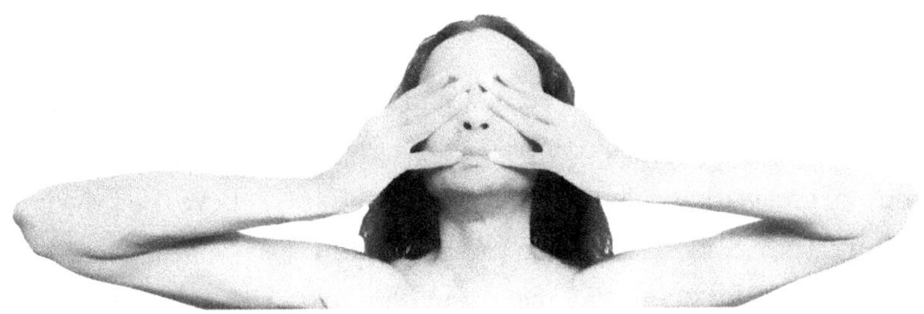

If you have learned a different hand position for this practice, then feel free to use that.

1. Exhale fully and close your eyes, concentrate on the Root FAP and inhale up the body with an ocean breath to the top AP (Crown BAP or Third Eye FAP) then apply your fingers on your face.
2. Exhale from your nose down the body with a humming sound to the Root FAP.
3. Remove your hands from your face before the start of the next round. Optionally, you may leave your hands on your face for the duration of the practice.

This completes 1 round. Perform rounds for 1 to 2 minutes.

Breath Meditation

Breath meditation involves sitting perfectly still and breathing silently with just a minimal movement of the diaphragm. It is during meditation when the most powerful spiritual experiences tend to happen. The way to enable this is to completely let go and open yourself up fully to all possibilities.

1. Once comfortable, make a firm commitment to remain perfectly still for the entire practice. Close your eyes and focus at the point between the entrance of your nostrils and feel your breath flowing in and out of your nostrils.
2. The goal is to have a perfectly equal flow of breath between the two nostrils. Move your concentration over to the opening of the less open nostril and wait as the flow increases. Once you believe the flow is equal, return your concentration to the center and observe if that is so.
3. Finally, just be open and accepting of all experiences that may occur. Continue for 5 minutes.

Daily Practice (13-15 min)

- Alternate Nostril Breathing (1-2 min)
- Kriya Breathing (6 min)
- Face Fingers Breathing (1-2 min)
- Breath Meditation (5 min)

If unable to do the practices in later lessons, or if simply not interested in them, you may increase this practice up to 1 hour if desired.

- Alternate Nostril Breathing (3 min)
- Kriya Breathing (24 min)
- Face Fingers Breathing (3 min)
- Breath Meditation (30 min)

Lesson 2: Basic Asana

This lesson introduces some simple physical postures and body movements, including a formal sitting posture and a kriya breathing practice, all still suitable for all ages, but feel free to skip or modify anything you are unable to do.

See the Daily Practice schedule for correctly ordering these practices with the ones from Lesson 1.

Lying Down Stretch

Lie down on your back, raise your hands up over your head, inhale deeply with your diaphragm and stretch your fingers up and your toes down. Hold for a few seconds, then relax, breathe and take another deep breath, hold and stretch a second time. Relax, breathe and bring your arms back down by your side.

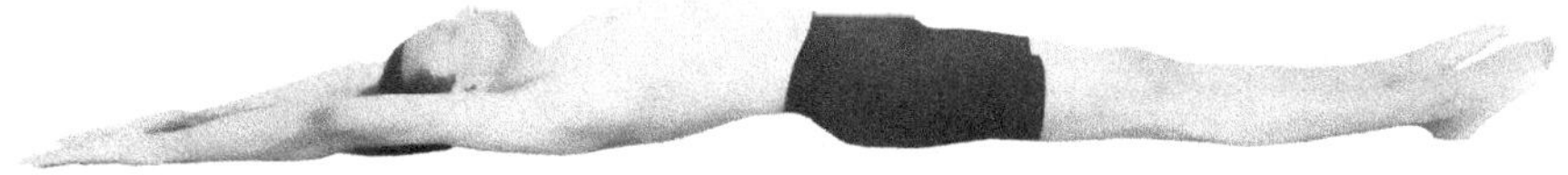

Lower Back Massage

While lying on your back, bend your knees and pull them toward your chest with your hands such that the lower back presses against the ground. Gently rock back and forth and side to side to allow every part of the lower back to press against the ground. If you're able to, touch your knees to your forehead then your chin and roll up to a sitting position. Otherwise, extend your legs, roll on your side and push yourself up to a sitting position.

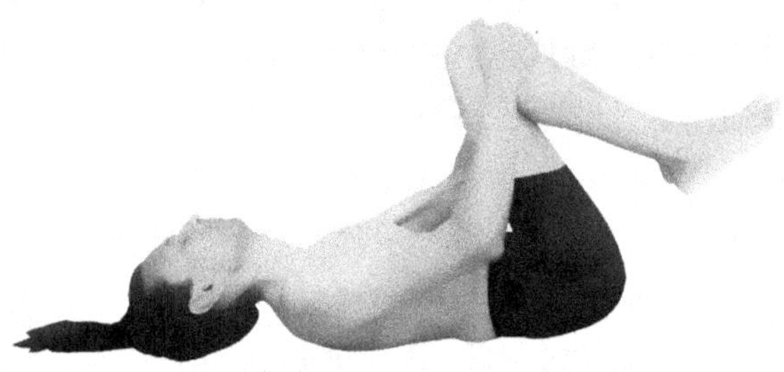

Ankle Rotation

While sitting on the ground, extend your legs with your feet apart. Point your toes down, rotate in, up, out and back down. Repeat in the other direction. Relax your feet and wiggle your toes for a few seconds.

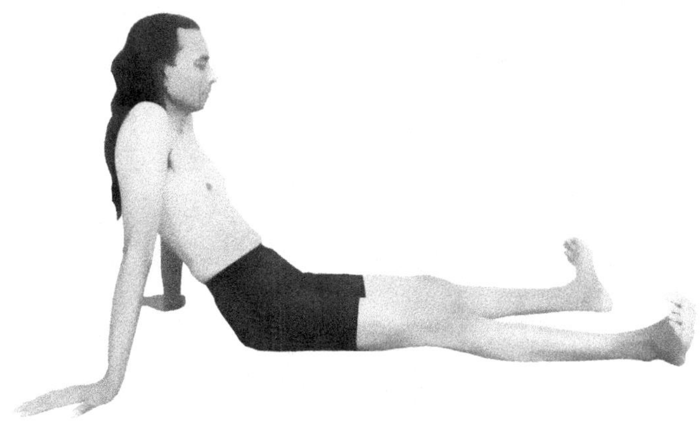

Squat Pose

From a sitting position come up on your feet in a squat with your feet flat on the ground. Squat down as low as you can and hold for a few seconds.

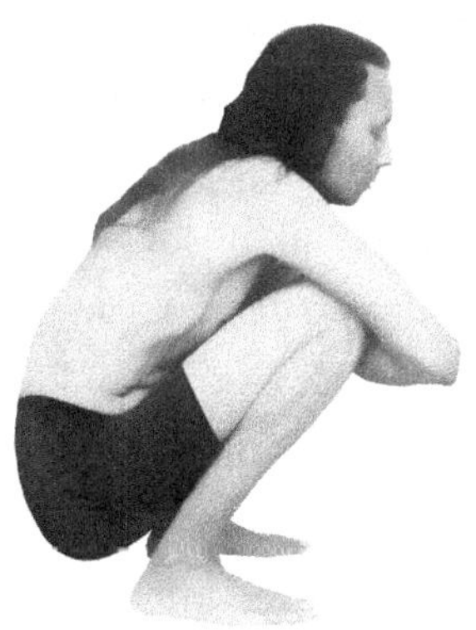

Tiptoe Pose

From the squat come up on your toes and try balancing with your hands in prayer pose and hold for a few seconds. Sit back down when done.

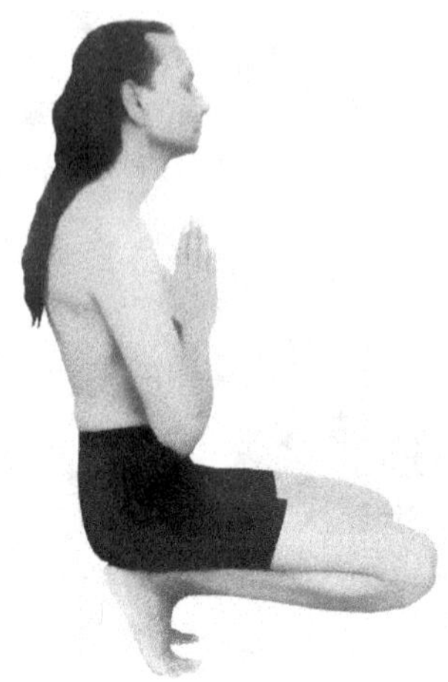

Accomplished Pose (siddhasana)

This is the recommended sitting posture for these practices, but any sitting posture on the ground is fine. It is also fine to use a cushion or rolled up blanket to raise yourself off the ground a bit to help relieve pressure from your legs. The main thing is to have your back straight by holding your head high and creating a slight inward curve at the lower back.

The Accomplished Pose is done with the legs crossed, then adjust your feet such that your heels are lined up one on top of the other with the lower heel pressed against the perineum/vulva area. Tuck your toes on both feet between the calf and thigh to create a stable and firm seat.

Check for the slight inward curve at the lower back and if not there you may have to raise yourself off the ground a bit until you have it. With daily practice the flexibility in your legs will improve, and one day you'll be able to sit comfortably directly on the ground.

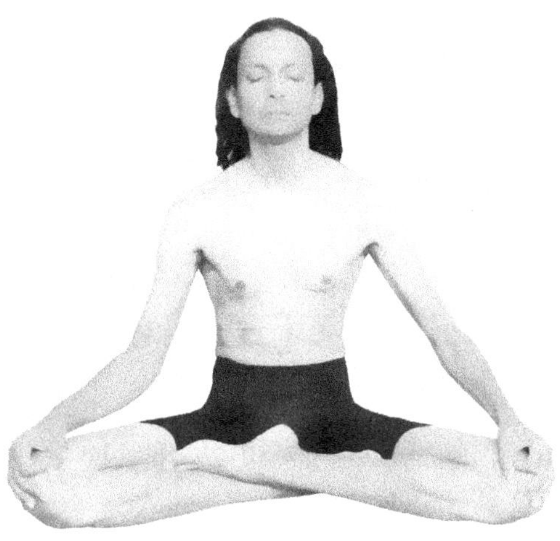

If you have learned a different way of sitting, then feel free to use that.

Hand Position

When sitting still for meditation, you can touch the tip of your thumb and index finger together and rest your hands on the knees with your fingers pointing down.

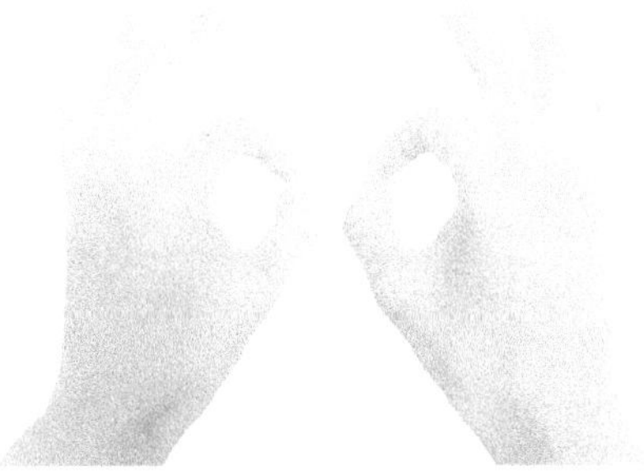

For a firmer position, you can also curl your index finger more, such that the top segment of your finger is pressed against the side of your thumb.

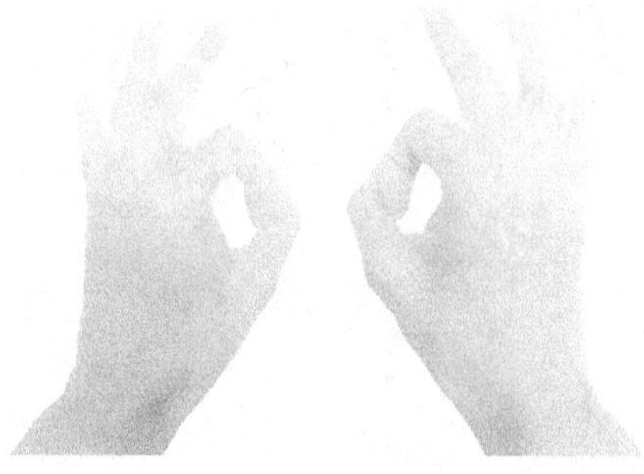

If you have learned a different hand position, then feel free to use that.

Forward Bending Breathing (maha mudra)

Forward bending breathing involves bending and extending the legs with ocean breathing. This practice purifies the entire network of spiritual pathways in the body and stimulates the flow of spiritual energy in the spine.

1. From your sitting posture, raise your right knee such that your right foot is flat on the ground, while your left leg remains where it is and your back remains straight. Use your hands or arms to pull your right thigh against your chest. Exhale fully and close your eyes, concentrate on the Root FAP and inhale up the body to the top AP (Crown BAP or Third Eye FAP).

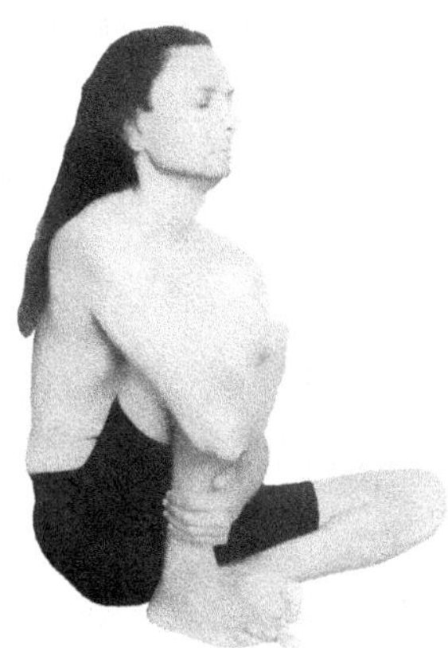

2. While concentrating on the top AP (Crown BAP or Third Eye FAP), exhale normally while extending your right leg straight and bending forward to hold your right foot.

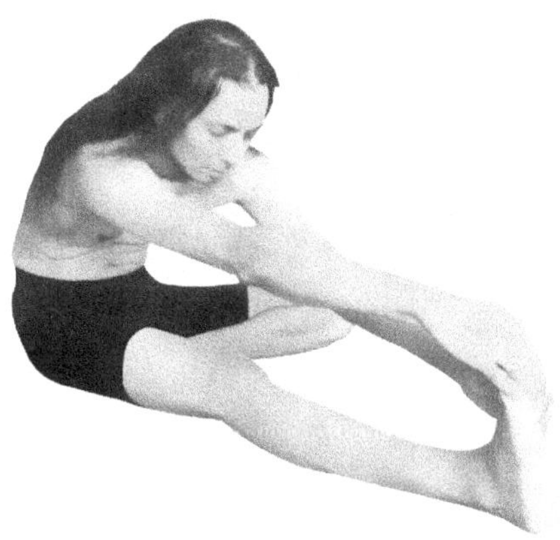

3. Inhale normally while sitting up straight and bending your right leg to return to the starting position in Step 1.
4. Concentrate on the top AP (Crown BAP or Third Eye FAP) and exhale down the body to the Root FAP.

5. Hold the air out while swapping leg positions, then repeat the practice with your left leg.

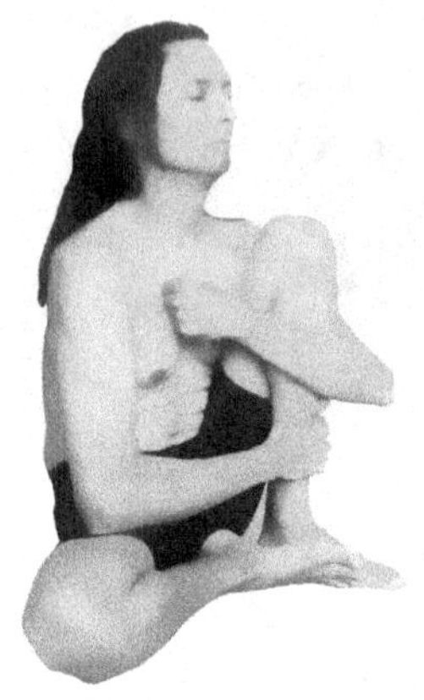

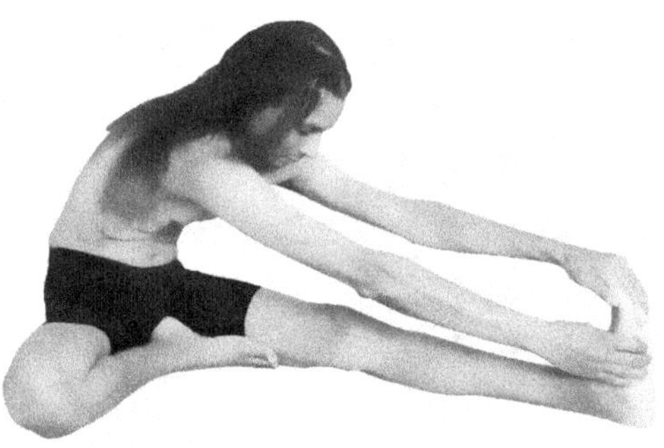

6. Hold the air out while bringing both legs up with knees bent, then repeat the practice with both legs.

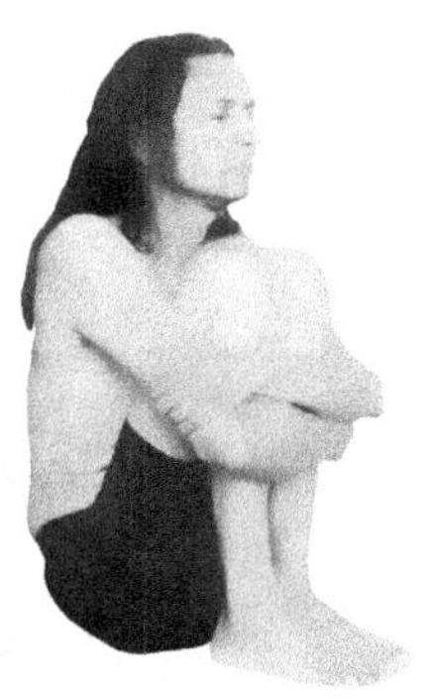

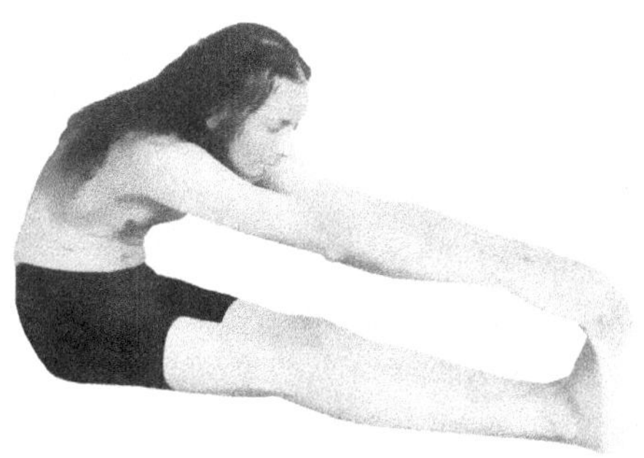

This completes 1 round. Perform rounds for 2 to 3 minutes.

Daily Practice (16-20 min)

Movements/Postures (1-2 min)

- Lying Down Stretch
- Lower Back Massage
- Ankle Rotation
- Squat Pose
- Tiptoe Pose

Kriyas/Breathing (10-13 min)

- Alternate Nostril Breathing (1-2 min)
- Kriya Breathing (6 min)
- Forward Bending Breathing (2-3 min)
- Face Fingers Breathing (1-2 min)

Meditation (5 min)

- Breath Meditation (5 min)

If unable to do the practices in later lessons, or if simply not interested in them, you can increase this practice up to 1 hour if desired.

- Movements/Postures (1-2 min)
- Alternate Nostril Breathing (1-2 min)
- Kriya Breathing (24 min)
- Forward Bending Breathing (2-3 min)
- Face Fingers Breathing (1-2 min)
- Breath Meditation (30 min)

Lesson 3: Intermediate Asana

This lesson introduces some more advanced physical postures and body movements, along with a more forceful breathing practice.

This is the point where the risk increases for the elderly, children under 12, those with health issues, pregnant women, etc. The two practices you may want to avoid if you fall into one of these categories is the Abdominal Lock and Rapid Belly Breathing. If in doubt, please check with your doctor before proceeding.

It's perfectly fine to skip these two practices or even just stick with the practices in Lessons 1 and/or 2, as this will still be a vast improvement over not having any spiritual practice. This is why I've provided the 1 hour option for each of those lessons.

See the Daily Practice schedule for correctly ordering these practices with the ones from previous lessons.

Sun Salutation (surya namaskar)

The sun salutation is the best way to revitalize the whole body to maximize the benefits of the kriya breathing and meditation practices that follow.

1. Standing with your hands in prayer pose, inhale and exhale.

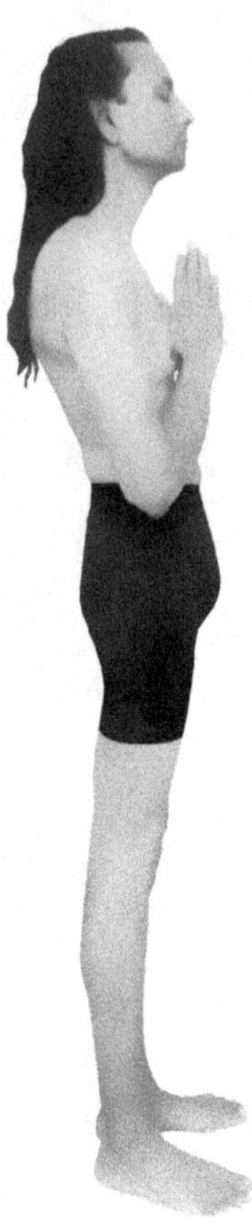

2. Inhale while stretching your hands up over your head and bending your body and arms backward about 45 degrees.

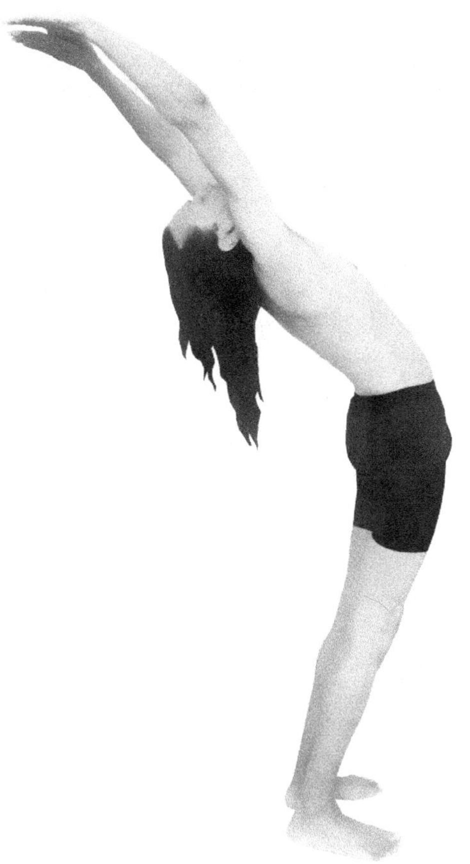

3. Exhale while bending forward and reaching down to touch your toes and ideally placing your palms flat on the ground next to your feet while keeping your knees straight.

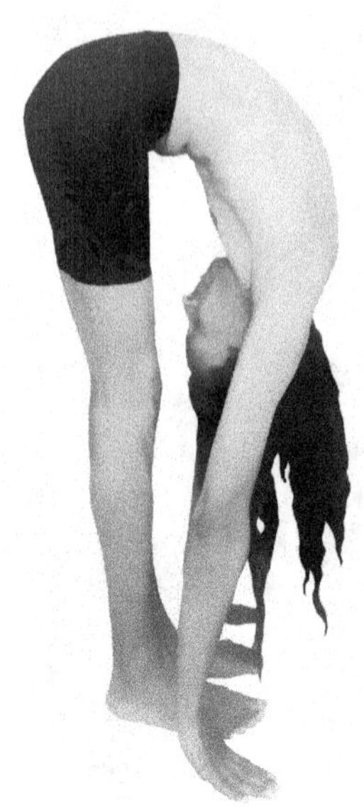

4. Inhale while squatting down and extending your right leg back with your toes pointed back. Lift your head up and back while your left foot remains flat and both palms too, ideally not moving from Step 3.

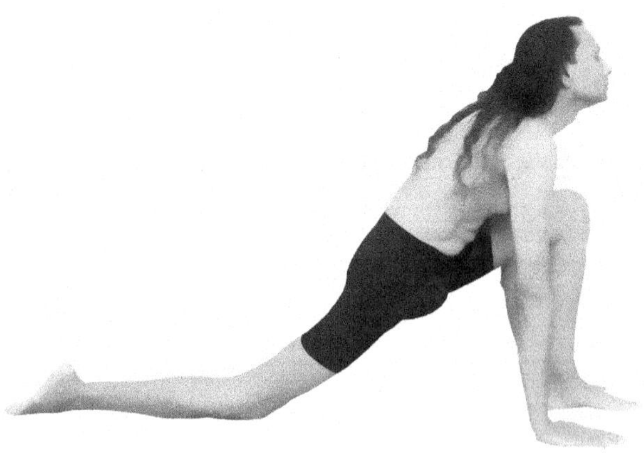

5. Exhale while bringing your left foot back and coming up on your knees, then come up on your toes and try to press your heels to the ground

while keeping your arms and legs straight. Ideally, palms not moving since Step 3.

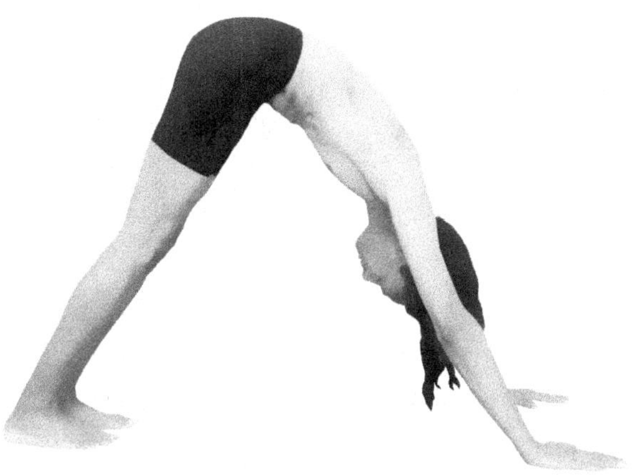

6. Hold the air out while bringing your head down to touch your nose, then chin, then chest, then knees to the ground while keeping your body compressed so your butt sticks up in the air. Ideally, palms not moving since Step 3.

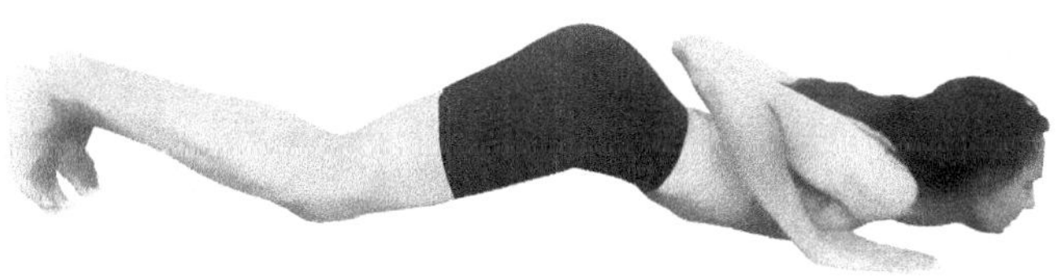

7. Lie flat, then inhale while pushing your upper body up and back with your arms, while also keeping your legs flat on the ground. Ideally, palms not moving since Step 3.

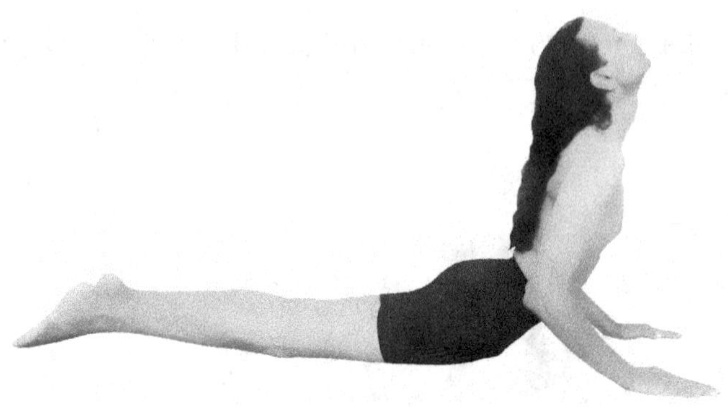

8. Exhale and lift your hips and legs off the ground then come up on your toes and try to press your heels to the ground while keeping your arms and legs straight. Same position as in Step 5. Ideally, palms not moving since Step 3.

9. Inhale and bring your left foot between your hands while extending your right leg back with your toes pointed back. Lift your head up and back. Same position as in Step 4. Ideally, palms not moving since Step 3.

10. Exhale and bring your right foot between your hands while straightening your knees. Same position as in Step 3. Ideally, palms not moving since Step 3.

11. Inhale and bring your hands up over your head while stretching up and bending your body and arms backward about 45 degrees. Same position as in Step 2.

12. Exhale while returning to a normal standing position with your hands in prayer pose. Same position as in Step 1.

Perform all 12 steps again, except with your left leg back in steps 4 and 9. If you have learned a different way of performing the Sun Salutation, then feel free to use that.

Corpse Pose

Lie down on your back and relax for a few seconds. Breathe deeply with the diaphragm until breathing returns to normal after the physical exertion of the Sun Salutation.

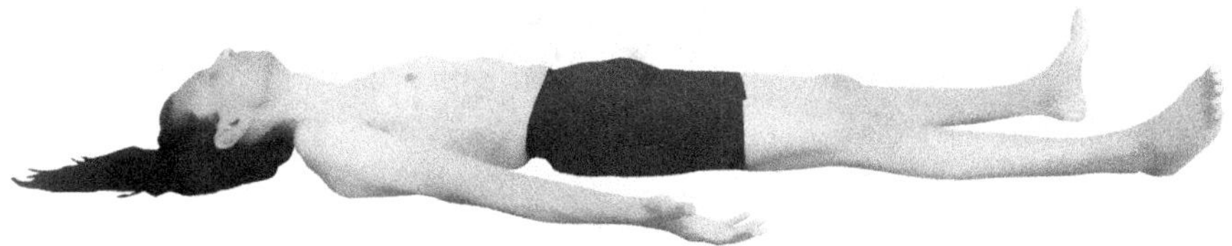

Spinal Twist

From a sitting position, raise the right knee such that the right foot is flat on the ground. Swivel the left leg, keeping it on the ground, such that the left knee is next to the right foot. Lift the right foot and place it on the other side of the left knee. Twist your body towards the raised right knee and wrap your left arm around it. Place your right hand on the ground behind you for stability and move your left arm to the other side of the right knee to twist the body further to the right. Hold your left knee with your left hand while twisting your head, shoulders and torso to the right as much as possible. Hold for a few seconds then repeat in the other direction.

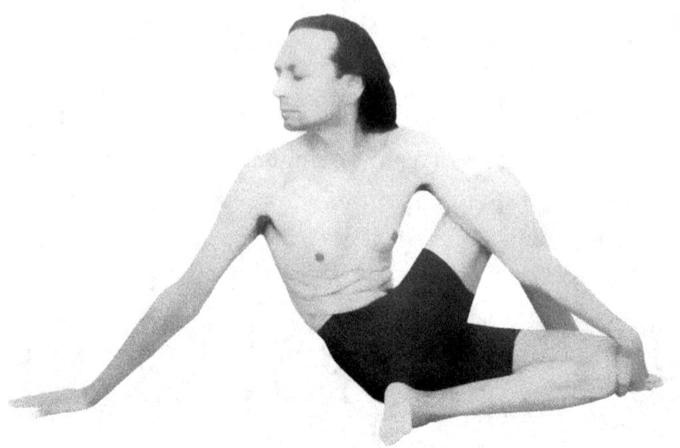

Abdominal Lock (uddiyana bandha)

From a standing position with your feet apart and knees bent, bend forward placing your hands just above your knees. Exhale fully and hold the air out, then pull your navel to the spine and your diaphragm up under the rib cage. Hold for a few seconds, then release and inhale. Take a few deep breaths to restore normal breathing.

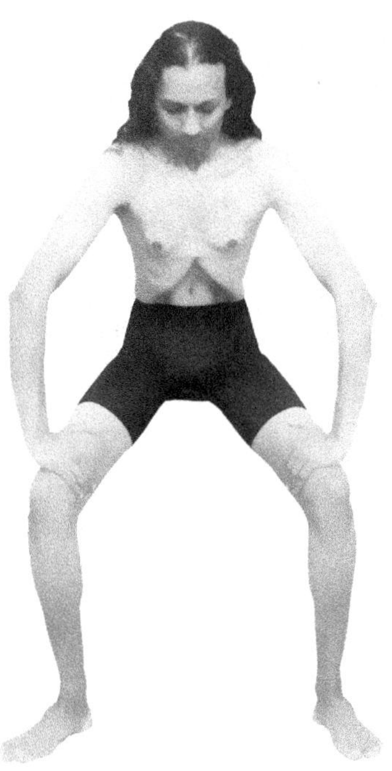

Rapid Belly Breathing (bhastrika)

Rapid belly breathing involves the continuous rapid expansion and contraction of the belly to force air in and out of the lungs. Within the spinal passage there are three spiritual knots (granthis) which need to be broken for kundalini energy to flow freely. This practice breaks those knots.

1. Inhale fully expanding your belly, then rapidly contract your belly forcing air out through your nose, then immediately expand your belly to suck air in through your nose.

This completes 1 round. Start with 10 rounds per practice, then increase to 20 rounds per practice. Each round should take about half a second, so 20 rounds should take about 10 seconds.

Daily Practice (21-26 min)

Movements/Postures (6-8 min)

- Sun Salutation
- Corpse Pose
- Lying Down Stretch (optional)
- Lower Back Massage
- Spinal Twist
- Ankle Rotation
- Squat Pose
- Tiptoe Pose
- Abdominal Lock

Kriyas/Breathing (10-13 min)

- Alternate Nostril Breathing (1-2 min)
- Rapid Belly Breathing (10 sec)
- Kriya Breathing (6 min)
- Forward Bending Breathing (2-3 min)
- Face Fingers Breathing (1-2 min)

Meditation (5 min)

- Breath Meditation (5 min)

If unable to do the practices in later lessons, or if simply not interested in them, you can increase this practice up to 1 hour if desired.

- Movements/Postures (6-8 min)
- Alternate Nostril Breathing (1-2 min)
- Rapid Belly Breathing (10 sec)
- Kriya Breathing (24 min)

- Forward Bending Breathing (2-3 min)
- Face Fingers Breathing (1-2 min)
- Breath Meditation (30 min)

Lesson 4: Intermediate Kriya

All spiritual practices may be categorized as being either passive or active. A passive practice will passively awaken the chakras and kundalini, while an active practice will actively awaken them.

The practices in Lessons 1 and 2 are entirely passive. Lesson 3 introduced two practices that lean toward the active side: the abdominal lock and rapid belly breathing. I gave a warning at the start of that lesson about this. This lesson introduces inner and outer breath retention which is very much an active practice and recommended only for those that are fit and healthy (physically, mentally and emotionally).

To know if you qualify for these practices, you should be able to read through this page on "Kundalini Syndrome"[7] which really just describes the normal and expected kundalini awakening experiences that may occur, and feel excited to experience them. One experience mentioned, which is highly sought after, is "Breathing spontaneously stopping." This is known as the breathless state (kevala kumbhaka) which will be discussed in later lessons.

Of course it's one thing to just read about these experiences and another to have them actually happen, so if you find yourself overwhelmed, just revert back to the passive practices until you can integrate the new level you've reached. Once you feel stable again, you can give the active practices another try.

---

[7] https://psychology.wikia.org/wiki/Kundalini_syndrome

Alternate Nostril Breathing (nadi shodhana)

This advanced version of the practice requires that you've reached the point where each inhale and exhale lasts for about 15 seconds. All previous instructions from Lesson 1 apply if not mentioned.

1. Exhale fully and close your eyes, then use your right thumb to close your right nostril and inhale fully through your left nostril for 15 seconds.
2. Hold your breath in for a few seconds.
3. Release your right nostril and use your middle and ring fingers to close your left nostril and exhale fully through your right nostril for 15 seconds.
4. Hold your breath out for a few seconds.
5. Keep your left nostril closed and inhale fully through your right nostril for 15 seconds.
6. Hold your breath in for a few seconds.
7. Release your left nostril and use your thumb to close your right nostril and exhale fully through your left nostril for 15 seconds.
8. Hold the breath out for a few seconds.
9. Release both nostrils and inhale up the body for 15 seconds.
10. Hold the breath in for a few seconds.
11. Exhale down the body for 15 seconds.
12. Hold the breath out for a few seconds.

This completes 1 round. The goal is to gradually increase your inner and outer breath retention until it is equal to each inhale and exhale. So if you inhale for 15 seconds, then hold the breath in for 15 seconds, exhale for 15 seconds and hold the breath out for 15 seconds.

At this point there is no need to keep your hand raised while holding your breath in and out. You can instead rest both hands on your knees during this time. This also gives you the option of using both hands for closing your nostrils, such that you use your right thumb to close your right nostril as usual, but now instead use your left thumb to close your left nostril for perfect symmetry. Of course, if you feel more comfortable using your right hand for both nostrils then certainly continue with that.

Rapid Belly Breathing (bhastrika)

This advanced version of the practice introduces single nostril breathing. All previous instructions from Lesson 3 apply if not mentioned.

1. Inhale fully expanding your belly and close your eyes to begin.
2. Close your right nostril using your right thumb and rapidly contract your belly forcing air out through your left nostril, then immediately expand your belly to suck air in through your left nostril. This completes 1 round. Perform 10 rounds.
3. Close your left nostril using your left thumb and repeat through your right nostril for 10 rounds.
4. Finally, leave both nostrils open and repeat for 10 rounds.

This completes the practice.

Kriya Breathing

This practice remains the same as it was given in Lesson 1, except the duration is increased from 6 to 12 minutes. If you're now able to have each inhale and exhale last about 15 seconds, then each round will take 30 seconds, so 24 rounds will be completed in 12 minutes.

Forward Bending Breathing (maha mudra)

This advanced version of the practice introduces inner breath retention during the forward bend. All previous instructions from Lesson 2 apply if not mentioned.

1. Same.

2. Hold the breath in and concentrate on the top AP (Crown BAP or Third Eye FAP) while extending your right leg straight and bending forward to hold your right foot.

3. After a few seconds begin sitting up straight and bending your right leg to return to the starting position in Step 1.

4. Same.

5. Same.

6. Same.

This completes 1 round. Perform one more round.

The goal is to gradually increase your inner breath retention until it is equal to each inhale and exhale. So if you inhale for 15 seconds, then hold the breath in for 15 seconds, and exhale for 15 seconds.

Face Fingers Breathing (bhramari)

This advanced version of the practice introduces inner breath retention when your fingers are on your face. The finger position is the same except now the ring fingers are pressing the nostrils closed. All previous instructions from Lesson 1 apply if not mentioned.

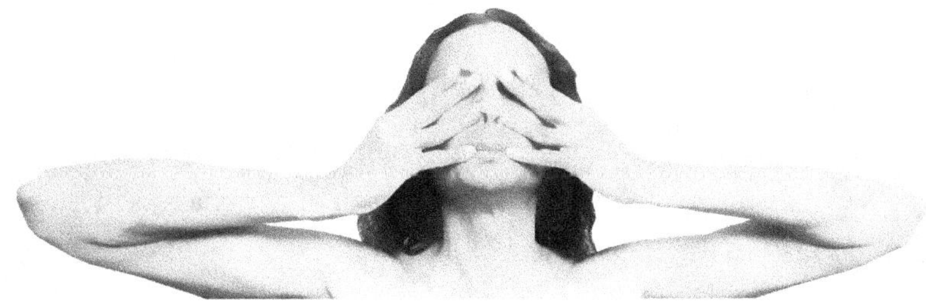

If you have learned a different hand position for this practice, then feel free to use that.

1. Exhale fully and close your eyes, concentrate on the Root FAP and inhale up the body to the top AP (Crown BAP or Third Eye FAP).

2. Hold your breath in, apply your fingers on your face, and concentrate on the Third Eye FAP. Continue holding for as long as comfortable, up to 1 minute.

3. When uncomfortable or at 1 minute, release just your ring fingers from your nostrils by moving them next to your middle fingers, and concentrate on the top AP (Crown BAP or Third Eye FAP).

4. Exhale from your nose, down the body with a humming sound to the Root FAP.

5. Remove your hands from your face before the start of the next round. Optionally, you may leave your hands on your face for the duration of the practice.

This completes 1 round. Perform one more round. The goal is to gradually increase your inner breath retention until it reaches 1 minute while paying attention to any sights or sounds that may appear.

Third Eye Meditation

Third Eye meditation is the same as the Breath meditation from Lesson 1 except our focus is now on the Third Eye FAP. This is the most direct method for actively awakening the Third Eye Chakra, which is necessary for developing psychic sensitivity to the chakras and the flow of spiritual energy in the body.

Kriya breathing becomes almost effortless when you are able to actually feel the spiritual energy flowing through your body and in your spine. You will also feel a distinct tingling sensation at each of the chakras in the spine and head along with tingling at their FAPs and BAPs. At night when sleeping, you may also experience lucid dreaming which is a great way to work through your emotional issues.

However, it's also important to not awaken advanced psychic abilities (telepathy, telekinesis, etc.) before you are ready for them, so I recommend alternating one month at a time between Third Eye and Breath meditation.

1. Once comfortable, make a firm commitment to remain perfectly still for the entire practice. Close your eyes and focus on the Third Eye FAP and feel the breath flowing in and out of that point.

2. Optionally, "Om" may be chanted mentally if desired. I recommend about once per second, and synchronized with the length of your inhale and exhale. For example, keep the length of the inhale and exhale the same at 4, 6 or 8 seconds and say the same number of Om's accordingly.

3. Finally, just be open and accepting of all experiences that may occur. Continue for 10 minutes.

Daily Practice (35-75 min)

Movements/Postures (6-10 min)

- Sun Salutation
- Corpse Pose
- Lying Down Stretch (optional)
- Lower Back Massage
- Spinal Twist
- Ankle Rotation
- Squat Pose
- Tiptoe Pose
- Abdominal Lock

Kriyas/Breathing (19-35 min)

- Alternate Nostril Breathing (2-3 min)
- Rapid Belly Breathing (15 sec)
- Kriya Breathing (12-24 min)
- Forward Bending Breathing (3-5 min)
- Face Fingers Breathing (2-3 min)

Meditation (10-30 min)

- Third Eye Meditation (10-30 min)

Lesson 5: Basic Locks

The final active practice is the lock (bandha or mudra) which is used to awaken a particular chakra or direct the flow of spiritual energy in the body. This lesson introduces four locks which will be incorporated into our practice.

Third Eye Lock (shambhavi mudra)

This lock is used to awaken the Third Eye Chakra.

Put your index finger in front of your face and look at the tip. Slowly move your finger towards the Third Eye FAP while following it with your eyes. When it touches the Third Eye FAP, look at the Third Eye FAP instead of your finger and move away your hand. Hold your eyes on the Third Eye FAP for a few seconds to apply the lock. Try maintaining the lock with your eyes closed and hold for a few more seconds, then relax your eyes to release the lock.

With practice, you will be able to focus directly on the Third Eye FAP without needing to use your index finger.

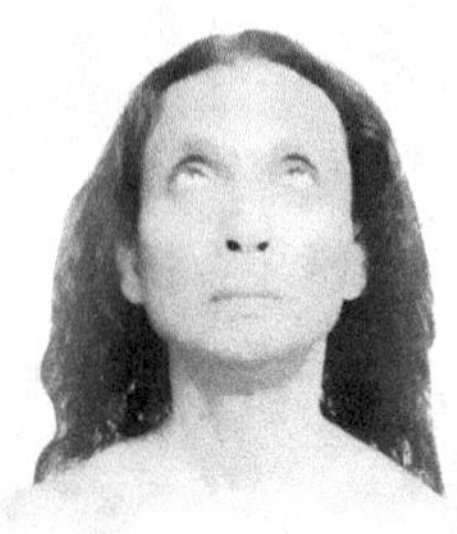

Nose Tip Lock (agochari mudra)

This is a secondary lock used to awaken the Root Chakra.

Put your index finger in front of your face and look at the finger tip. Slowly move your finger towards the tip of your nose while following it with your eyes. When it touches the nose tip, look at the nose tip instead of your finger and move away your hand. Hold your eyes on the nose tip for a few seconds to apply the lock. Try maintaining the lock with your eyes closed and hold for a few more seconds, then relax your eyes to release the lock.

With practice, you will be able to focus directly on the nose tip without needing to use your index finger.

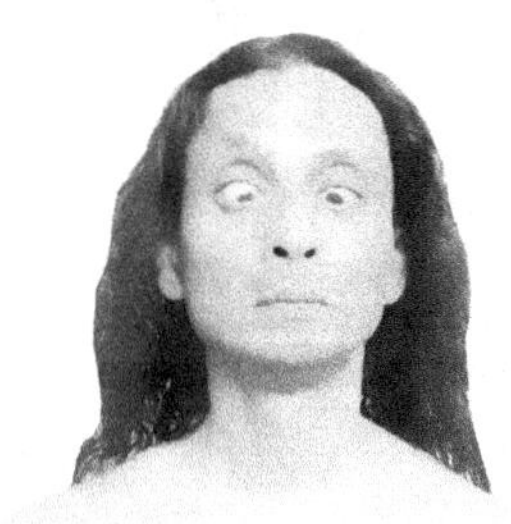

Basic Tongue Lock (khechari mudra - basic)

This lock is used to awaken the Palate Chakra and redirect energy from the tongue back into the body. This is the basic version of the lock. An advanced version will be given in Lesson 7.

Take the tip of your tongue and slide it back across the roof of your mouth towards the uvula as far back as it will go then hold it there. Press the underside of your tongue against the soft palate. Concentrate on where the tongue is pressing the soft palate to awaken the Palate Chakra. Hold for a few seconds to apply the lock, then relax your mouth and tongue to release the lock.

Root Lock (mula bandha)

This is the primary lock used to awaken the Root Chakra. Contract the muscles at the Root FAP (perineum/cervix) to apply the lock and hold for a few seconds. Relax those muscles to release it.

This lock is closely related to the Sacral Lock in Lesson 6 and the Anal Lock (ashwini mudra). To become familiar with the muscles in this part of the body, Kegel Exercises[8] are recommended.

Alternate Nostril Breathing (nadi shodhana)

The duration of each inhale, hold in, exhale, and hold out is given as 15 seconds, but feel free to use any duration you are comfortable with. All previous instructions apply if not mentioned.

1. Apply the Third Eye Lock, Tongue Lock and Root Lock. Try to hold these locks until instructed otherwise.
2. Exhale fully and close your eyes, then use your right thumb to close your right nostril and inhale fully through your left nostril for 15 seconds

---

[8]   https://www.healthline.com/health/kegel-exercises

with concentration on the Third Eye FAP.

3. Release your right nostril, move your hand to your knee and hold your breath in for 15 seconds.

4. During this time, open your eyes and cycle your concentration from the Third Eye FAP to the Tongue to the Root FAP and tighten each lock as you move to it. Optionally, you may mentally chant "Om" at each, or "Third Eye", "Tongue", "Root", or "Shambhavi", "Khechari", "Mul".

5. Switch from the Third Eye Lock to the Nose Tip Lock and close your eyes. Use your left thumb to close your left nostril and exhale fully through your right nostril for 15 seconds with concentration on the Nose Tip.

6. Release your left nostril, move your hand to your knee and hold your breath out for 15 seconds.

7. During this time, open your eyes and cycle your concentration from the Nose Tip to the Tongue to the Root FAP and tighten each lock as you move to it. Optionally, you may mentally chant "Om" at each, or "Nose Tip", "Tongue", "Root", or "Agochari", "Khechari", "Mul".

8. Switch from the Nose Tip Lock to the Third Eye Lock and close your eyes. Use your left thumb to close your left nostril and inhale fully through your right nostril for 15 seconds with concentration on the Third Eye FAP.

9. Release your left nostril, move your hand to your knee and hold your breath in for 15 seconds.

10. Repeat Step 4.

11. Repeat Step 5 except with the right nostril closed.

12. Repeat Step 6 with right nostril.

13. Repeat Step 7.

14. Switch from the Nose Tip Lock to the Third Eye Lock and close your eyes. Concentrate on the Root FAP and inhale fully through both nostrils up the body for 15 seconds, then hold your breath in for 15 seconds.

15. Repeat Step 4.

16. Switch from the Third Eye Lock to the Nose Tip Lock and close your eyes. Concentrate on the top AP (Crown BAP or Third Eye FAP) and

exhale fully through both nostrils down the body for 15 seconds, then hold your breath out for 15 seconds.

17. Repeat Step 7.

This completes 1 round. Optionally, you may do additional rounds up to a maximum of 12.

Rapid Belly Breathing (bhastrika)

All previous instructions apply if not mentioned.

1. Apply the Third Eye Lock, Tongue Lock and Root Lock. Try to hold these locks for the duration of the practice.
2. The rest of the practice is the same as Lesson 4.

This completes the practice. Optionally, you may increase the number of rounds from 10 to 20.

Kriya Breathing

All previous instructions apply if not mentioned.

1. Apply the Third Eye Lock, Tongue Lock and Root Lock. Try to hold these locks for the duration of the practice.
2. The rest of the practice is the same as Lesson 4 with each inhale and exhale lasting 15 seconds.

Perform a total of 24 rounds in about 12 minutes. Optionally, you may continue increasing the number of rounds by 12 from 24 to 36 to 48 up to a maximum of 108.

You can also continue to use your hands to count, even for 108 rounds. On your left hand continue counting individual rounds up to 12 rounds, then on your right hand count completed sets of 12 rounds. So after 3 fingers on the right hand (9 segments) you would've completed 108 rounds (12 x 9 = 108).

With 15 second inhales and exhales, 108 rounds will take 54 minutes. You goal should now be to elongate the inhales and exhales to 30 seconds, such that only 54 rounds will take 54 minutes. This leads to the breathless state (kevala kumbhaka) and kundalini awakening.

Forward Bending Breathing (maha mudra)

All previous instructions apply if not mentioned.

1. From your sitting posture, raise your right knee such that your right foot is flat on the ground, while your left leg remains where it is and your back remains straight. Use your hands or arms to pull your right thigh against your chest.
2. Apply the Third Eye Lock, Tongue Lock and Root Lock. Try to hold these locks for the duration of the practice.
3. Exhale fully and close your eyes, concentrate on the Root FAP and inhale up the body to the top AP (Crown BAP or Third Eye FAP) for 15 seconds.
4. Hold your breath in and concentrate on the top AP (Crown BAP or Third Eye FAP) while extending your right leg straight and bending forward to hold your right foot. Maintain this position for 15 seconds.
5. During this time, open your eyes and cycle your concentration from the Third Eye FAP to the Tongue to the Root FAP and tighten each lock as you move to it. Optionally, you may mentally chant "Om" at each, or "Third Eye", "Tongue", "Root", or "Shambhavi", "Khechari", "Mul".
6. Begin sitting up straight and bending your right leg to return to the starting position in Step 1. Concentrate on the top AP (Crown BAP or Third Eye FAP) and exhale down the body to the Root FAP for 15 seconds.
7. Hold the air out while swapping leg positions, then repeat the practice with your left leg.
8. Hold the air out while bringing both legs up with knees bent, then repeat the practice with both legs.

This completes 1 round. Perform one more round. Optionally, you may do additional rounds up to a maximum of 12.

Face Fingers Breathing (bhramari)

All previous instructions apply if not mentioned.

1. Apply the Third Eye Lock, Tongue Lock and Root Lock. Try to hold these locks for the duration of the practice.
2. Exhale fully and close your eyes, concentrate on the Root FAP and inhale up the body to the top AP (Crown BAP or Third Eye FAP) for 15 seconds.
3. Hold your breath in, apply your fingers on your face, and concentrate on the Third Eye FAP. Continue holding your breath in for 1 minute.
4. During this time, you may concentrate exclusively on the Third Eye FAP or cycle your concentration from the Third Eye FAP to the Tongue to the Root FAP and tighten each lock as you move to it. Optionally, you may mentally chant "Om" at each, or "Third Eye", "Tongue", "Root", or "Shambhavi", "Khechari", "Mul".
5. Release just your ring fingers from your nostrils by moving them next to your middle fingers, and concentrate on the top AP (Crown BAP or Third Eye FAP).
6. Exhale from your nose, down the body with a humming sound to the Root FAP.
7. Remove your hands from your face before the start of the next round. Optionally, you may leave your hands on your face for the duration of the practice.

This completes 1 round. Perform one more round. Optionally, you may do additional rounds up to a maximum of 12.

Chakra Meditation

Chakra meditation refers to mediation on the Chakra FAPs. In Lesson 4 we introduced the Third Eye meditation, next would be to add the Heart FAP and then the Throat FAP, each for one month as part of our rotation with the Third Eye FAP and Breath meditations. You may also try the practice with the lower Chakra FAPs as well if you wish.

Meditation on the Heart FAP will help resolve all of your emotional issues such that you are able to remain in a state of joy, bliss, happiness and love most of the time, regardless of external circumstances.

Meditation on the Throat FAP will allow your diet to naturally move to lighter and lighter foods. You will first lose your taste for red meat and then all meat. You may even move away from eggs and dairy to a completely plant based diet. Just let your intuition be your guide.

At some point you'll feel you're ready to discard the chakra meditations entirely. Your focus will again return to the Breath meditation and balancing the air flow in both nostrils. It is both the first and last meditation practice, for when the air flow is balanced, the breath leaves the left (ida) and right (pingala) nostrils and enters the spine (sushumna). This results in the breathless state (kevala kumbhaka) and kundalini awakening.

Daily Practice (35-75 min)

The same as Lesson 4 with the locks added.

Lesson 6: Intermediate Locks

This lesson introduces four more locks which will be incorporated into our practice.

Throat Lock (jalandhara bandha)

This lock is used to awaken the Throat Chakra.

Bend your head forward with slight pressure while keeping your back straight and hold for a few seconds to apply the lock. Relax your head and raise it back up to release the lock.

The point of concentration is the Throat FAP, but that is usually not used when combined with other locks.

Solar Lock (uddiyana bandha - breath out)

This lock is used to awaken the Solar Chakra.

Exhale fully and hold the breath out. Pull your navel to the spine and pull your diaphragm up under the rib cage. Hold for a few seconds while concentrating on the Solar FAP to apply the lock. Note that the Solar FAP is also pulled with the diaphragm under the rib cage. Relax your abdomen and inhale to release the lock.

This lock will be combined with the Throat Lock and added during Alternate Nostril Breathing.

Navel Lock (uddiyana bandha - breath in)

This lock is used to awaken the Navel Chakra.

Inhale fully into your belly with only your diaphragm and do not expand your chest. Hold your breath in and pull your navel to the spine, pushing the air up into your chest. Hold for a few seconds while concentrating on the Navel FAP to apply the lock. Relax your abdomen and exhale to release the lock.

This lock will be combined with the Throat Lock and added during Forward Bending Breathing.

Sacral Lock (vajroli/sahajoli mudra)

This lock is used to awaken the Sacral Chakra.

Contract the two urethral sphincter muscles. These are the muscles used to stop the flow of urine. Hold for a few seconds while concentrating on the Sacral FAP to apply the lock. Relax those muscles to release the lock. This lock will be added during Face Fingers Breathing.

Alternate Nostril Breathing (nadi shodhana)

The Throat Lock and Solar Lock are now added when holding your breath out during Step 7. All previous instructions apply if not mentioned.

Replace Step 7 with the following:

- During this time, open your eyes and apply the Throat Lock and Solar Lock. Cycle your concentration from the Nose Tip to the Solar FAP to the Root FAP and tighten each lock as you move to it. Optionally, you may mentally chant "Om" at each, or "Nose Tip", "Solar", "Root", or "Agochari", "Uddiyana", "Mul". At the end of the time release the Throat Lock and Solar Lock.

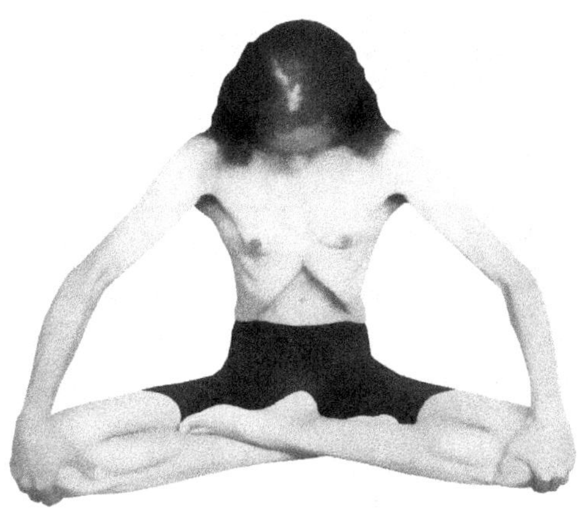

Forward Bending Breathing (maha mudra)

The Throat Lock and Navel Lock are now added when holding your breath in during Step 5. All previous instructions apply if not mentioned.
Replace Step 5 with the following:

- During this time, open your eyes and apply the Throat Lock and Navel Lock. Cycle your concentration from the Third Eye FAP to the Navel FAP to the Root FAP and tighten each lock as you move to it. Optionally, you may mentally chant "Om" at each, or "Third Eye", "Navel", "Root", or "Shambhavi", "Uddiyana", "Mul". At the end of the time release the Throat Lock and Navel Lock.

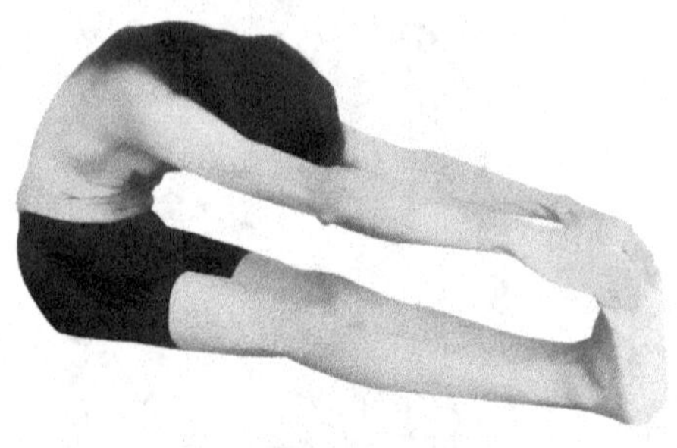

Face Fingers Breathing (bhramari)

The Sacral Lock is now added when holding your breath in during Step 4. All previous instructions apply if not mentioned.

Replace Step 4 with the following:

- During this time, apply the Sacral Lock. You may concentrate exclusively on the Third Eye FAP or cycle your concentration from the Third Eye FAP to the Sacral FAP to the Root FAP and tighten each lock as you move to it. Optionally, you may mentally chant "Om" at each, or "Third Eye", "Sacral", "Root", or "Shambhavi", "Vajroli/Sahajoli", "Mul". At the end of the time release the Sacral Lock.

Daily Practice (35-75 min)

The same as Lesson 5 with the locks added.

Lesson 7: Advanced Tongue Lock

The final lock to learn is the Advanced Tongue Lock which requires the ability to insert the tongue into the nasopharynx[9]. To develop this ability requires lengthening the skin under the tongue that attaches it to the base of the mouth. This piece of skin is called the frenulum. By first learning to click your tongue, you can then learn how to stretch and lengthen the frenulum, and finally achieve the Advanced Tongue Lock.

Tongue Clicking

Open your mouth slightly and press your tongue against the roof of your mouth. Create some suction to hold your tongue against the roof of your mouth, then pull it away such that it snaps against the floor of your mouth creating a clicking noise. Repeat 5 times.

This practice may be discontinued once the Advanced Tongue Lock has been achieved.

Frenulum Stretch

Open your mouth slightly and press your tongue against the roof of your mouth. Create some suction to hold your tongue against the roof of your mouth, then open your mouth wide to stretch the frenulum and hold for a

---

[9] https://upload.wikimedia.org/wikipedia/commons/2/2e/
     Blausen_0872_UpperRespiratorySystem.png

few seconds. Repeat 10 times.

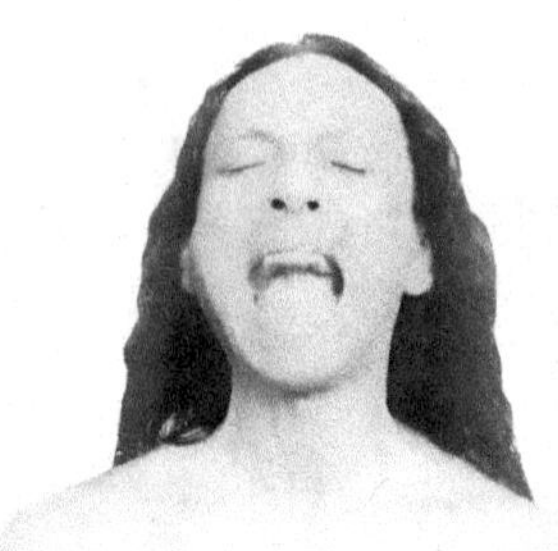

You should feel the frenulum being stretched, but if you make it sore, skip this practice until it heals and then continue. Also, this practice may be discontinued once the Advanced Tongue Lock has been achieved.

Full Face Stretch

Apply the Third Eye Lock, open the mouth wide and stretch the tongue out and down toward the chin. Hold for a few seconds then relax the face.

Not only do we stretch the tongue in this practice, but all of the facial muscles as well, so this one is good to continue even after the Advanced Tongue Lock has been achieved.

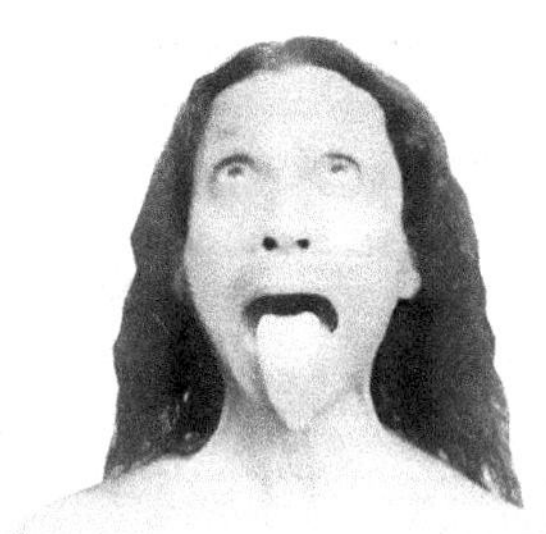

Advanced Tongue Lock (khechari mudra - advanced)

This lock redirects energy from your tongue into the Third Eye Chakra, and closes a spiritual circuit that connects your spine to your brain. This helps to achieve the breathless state (kevala kumbhaka) and kundalini awakening.

After some time of practicing the Frenulum Stretch and the Basic Tongue Lock, the tip of your tongue will be able to reach back and almost touch the uvula. When this happens, the Advanced Tongue Lock may be attempted by using your index and middle fingers to press against the base of your tongue such that the tip enters the nasopharynx. Once this happens, quickly push your tongue into the nasopharynx as far as it will go. Remove your fingers and try to hold your tongue there.

Initially, a lot of saliva will be produced, and your tongue will slip back out into your mouth fairly quickly, but with continued daily practice the saliva will reduce, and your tongue will be able to stay longer in the nasopharynx. At some point no saliva will be produced and your tongue will be able to rest comfortably on the floor of the nasopharynx with the tip touching the base of the nasal septum.

Initially, try keeping your tongue here on the floor of the nasopharynx touching the base of the nasal septum for the entire duration of your yoga practice, including postures, breathing and meditation. The point of concentration is where the tip of your tongue is pressing.

For the final position, keep most of your tongue on the floor of the nasopharynx, then stretch the tip up and press it into the corner where the top of the nasal septum meets the roof of the nasopharynx. This is the final position used for your entire yoga practice.

Next, turn your tongue sideways and try inserting it into your left and right nostrils. Verify you can fully block the air flow for one nostril while keeping the other fully open. This can now be used for Alternate Nostril Breathing and Rapid Belly Breathing allowing the hands to remain on the knees.

Additionally, on the left and right side of the nasopharynx you will find the opening of the eustachian tubes connecting to the left and right ears. These and many other areas in the nasopharynx benefit from being pressed by the tongue, so give the whole area a massage with your tongue. This can be done daily just before starting your yoga practice.

Eventually, you will no longer need to use your fingers to push your tongue in, as your tongue will be able to enter the nasopharynx on its own.

Kriya Breathing

If you have so far been using "down the spine" breathing for chakra awakening, and you've developed sensitivity to the flow of energy in your body and the chakras, then you may now want to try "up the spine" breathing for kundalini awakening. You can introduce this by splitting your practice in two. Continue with "down the spine" for Alternate Nostril Breathing and the first 12 rounds or 6 minutes of Kriya Breathing, then switch to "up the spine" for the last 12 rounds or 6 minutes of Kriya Breathing as well as Forward Bending Breathing and Face Fingers Breathing.

Once you develop sensitivity to the flow of energy up the spine, you may switch your entire practice to "up the spine" breathing for kundalini awakening.

Daily Practice Summary

Movements/Postures

1. Sun Salutation
2. Corpse Pose
3. Lying Down Stretch (optional)
4. Lower Back Massage
5. Spinal Twist
6. Ankle Rotation
7. Squat Pose
8. Tiptoe Pose
9. Abdominal Lock

Advanced Tongue Lock Preparation

1. Tongue Clicking
2. Frenulum Stretch
3. Full Face Stretch
4. Advanced Tongue Lock (with fingers)

Alternate Nostril Breathing

1. Apply the Third Eye Lock (eyes closed), Tongue Lock and Root Lock.
2. Inhale left nostril with concentration at Third Eye FAP.
3. Hold breath in, open eyes, cycle from Third Eye FAP to Tongue to Root FAP.
4. Apply the Nose Tip Lock (eyes closed).
5. Exhale right nostril with concentration at Nose Tip.
6. Hold breath out, open eyes, apply Throat Lock and Solar Lock, cycle from Nose Tip to Solar FAP to Root FAP.
7. Repeat steps 1-3 with right nostril.
8. Repeat steps 4-6 with left nostril.
9. Repeat steps 1-3 with both nostrils up the body.
10. Repeat steps 4-6 with both nostrils down the body.

Rapid Belly Breathing

1. Apply the Third Eye Lock (eyes closed), Tongue Lock and Root Lock.
2. Perform 10 rapid belly breaths with left nostril.
3. Repeat with the right nostril then both nostrils.

Kriya Breathing

1. Apply the Third Eye Lock (eyes closed), Tongue Lock and Root Lock.
2. Inhale up the body then exhale down the body.
3. Repeat step 2 for 24 times.

Forward Bending Breathing

1. Apply the Third Eye Lock (eyes closed), Tongue Lock and Root Lock.
2. Right leg up, inhale up the body.
3. Hold breath in, right leg out forward bend, open eyes, apply Throat Lock and Navel Lock, cycle from Third Eye FAP to Navel FAP to Root FAP.
4. Right leg up, exhale down the body.
5. Repeat with the left leg then both legs.
6. Repeat all steps a second time.

Face Fingers Breathing

1. Apply the Third Eye Lock (eyes closed), Tongue Lock and Root Lock.
2. Inhale up the body, hold the breath in, apply fingers on face and Sacral Lock.
3. Concentrate on Third Eye FAP or cycle from Third Eye FAP to Sacral FAP to Root FAP.
4. Release nostril fingers, exhale down the body with a humming sound.
5. Repeat all steps a second time.

Chakra/Breath Meditation

1. Sit still, close eyes, concentrate on chakra FAP or breath at nostril entrance.

Conclusion

Thank you for taking the time to read my book on Kriya Yoga! I hope you found it useful.

Having a daily spiritual practice is the first step in your journey of truly understanding what it means to be a human being. As your awareness expands you will likely have many questions and want to deepen your understanding of spirituality. I've created a site on Patreon[10] to help you do just that.

I launched my Patreon site on May 19, 2020 with a 24 hour $1/month subscription sale. I had 15 people sign up at that price and some even offered more. I'm extremely grateful for their support and this book may not have happened without them. So in celebration of this book becoming a reality, I've decided to offer unlimited subscriptions priced at $1/month for the time being.

At launch, I live streamed lessons that were the basis for this book. Subscribers are able to review those video lessons whenever they wish, as well as attend weekly live group sessions. On May 2, 2021, I'll once again begin live streamed classes on the updated lessons as they are presented in this book. If you're reading this after that date, the recorded videos will be available for viewing.

I'm extremely thrilled that you've read my book and thank you so much for doing so.

All my love and gratitude,

---

[10] https://www.patreon.com/ManojTheYogi

Manoj the Yogi

Recommended Reading

"Art of Super-Realization: Initiation"[11] by Paramahansa Yogananda

"Kundalini Tantra"[12] by Swami Satyananda Saraswati

"A Systematic Course In The Ancient Tantric Techniques Of Yoga And Kriya"[13] by Swami Satyananda Saraswati

"Hatha Yoga Pradipika"[14] by Swami Muktibodhananda Saraswati

"Mastering Pranayama: From Breathing Techniques to Kundalini Awakening"[15] by Radhika Shah Grouven.

[11] https://www.goodreads.com/book/show/26823823-art-of-super-realization

[12] https://www.goodreads.com/book/show/137527.Kundalini_Tantra

[13] https://www.goodreads.com/book/show/1037866.A_Systematic_Course
_In_The_Ancient_Tantric_Techniques_Of_Yoga_And_Kriya

[14] https://www.goodreads.com/book/show/199514.Hatha_Yoga_Pradipika

[15] https://www.goodreads.com/book/show/39901949-mastering-pranayama

About the Author

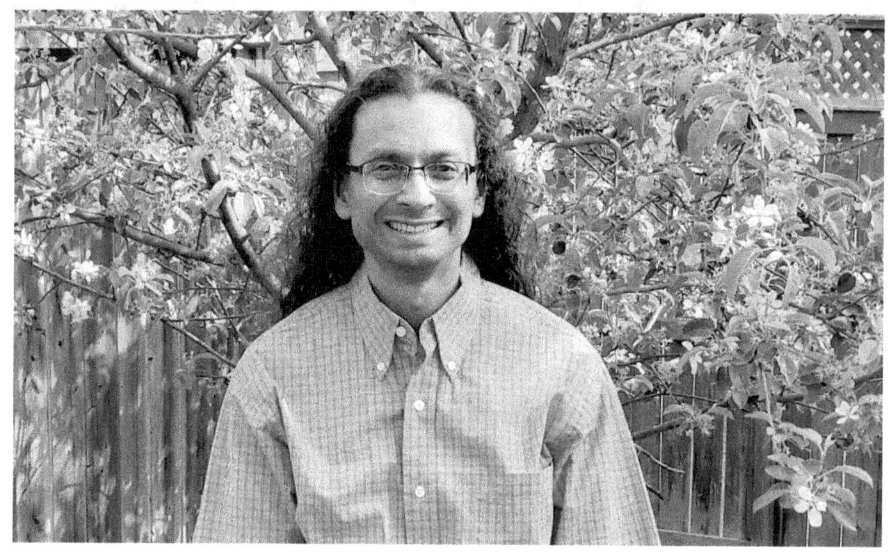

My Apple Tree and I

Manoj Prasad began a disciplined yoga practice on November 1, 2001 which led to a variety of spiritual experiences. In 2007, he began giving yoga classes to family and friends. Starting in 2011, videos of these classes were posted on YouTube at the "Manoj the Yogi"[16] channel. As of November 1, 2020, his channel has over 750,000 views, over 30,000 hours watched and over 7,600 subscribers.

Manoj was born in 1964, in London, UK, but grew up in Regina, Saskatchewan, Canada. He has been married to his wife Vini sine 1988,

---

[16] https://www.youtube.com/user/ManojTheYogi

and they have raised 3 adult children together. They have all been living in Ottawa, Canada since 2006. Manoj has degree in Electrical Engineering and has worked as a Software Developer for his entire career.

In 2020, Manoj launched a Patreon[17] site and wrote a book on Kriya Yoga to begin growing his fledgling career as a yogi.

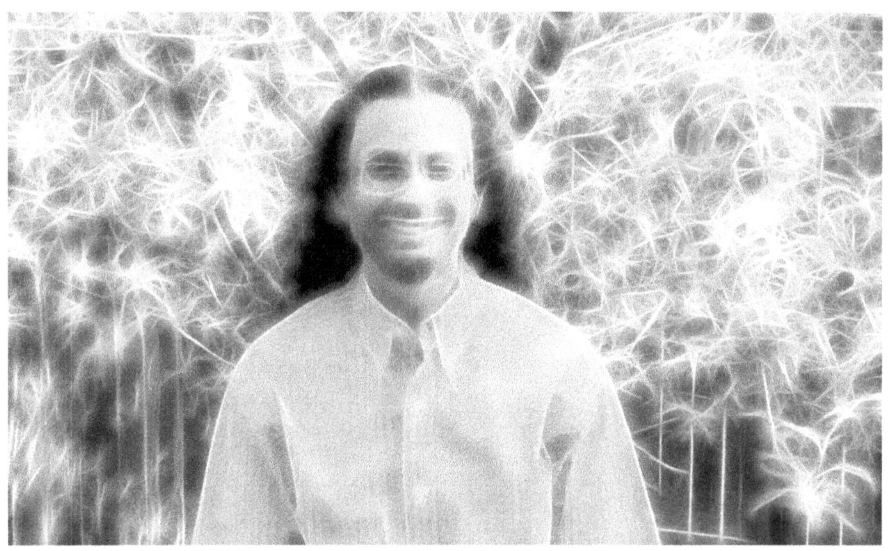

...in the Spirit World

---

[17] https://www.patreon.com/ManojTheYogi